M000239670

ADAM HELLER'S

ZERO PAIN NOW

WORKBOOK

ADAM HELLER'S
ZERO PAIN NOW

Published and distributed by Mirelle Publishing, LLC.

Adam Heller's *Zero Pain Now* Process
Copyright © 2011 by Adam Heller

All rights reserved. No part of this book may be reproduced or transmitted in any form, or by any means, including but not limited to, any mechanical, photographic, or electronic process. Nor may it be stored in a retrieval system, transmitted, or otherwise copied for public or private use without written permission from the publisher.

First Edition: August, 2011
10 9 8 7 6 5 4 3 2 1

For bulk purchases of this book, please contact the publisher:
Special Markets, Mirelle Publishing, LLC.
P.O. Box 4948 - Laguna Beach, CA 92652

Visit our website: www.zeropainnow.com
Phone: 949-497-8383
Email: info@zeropainnow.com

ISBN: 978-0-9839107-2-5

Printed in the United States of America

Cover Design by: Maria Janosko

READ THIS FIRST

The author of this book does not dispense medical advice or prescribe any technique as a form of treatment for medical problems. The intent of the author is to offer information of a general nature to help the reader in their quest to heal psychologically caused physical pain. This book is not to be used as a substitute for a medical diagnosis or medical treatment.

If you are experiencing physical pain, you must see a doctor to rule out the possibility of a serious medical illness. All efforts have been made to assure the accuracy of the information contained in this book as of the publication date. The author and the publisher assume no responsibility for any actions of the reader as a result of applying these methods.

WELCOME

Welcome to the *Zero Pain Now* companion workbook. I've designed this workbook to help you accelerate your process of becoming free of pain and other symptoms.

The questions, tips and resources included here will help you better understand the real cause of your pain. In addition, doing the daily exercises will enable you to free yourself from limiting pain and get back to the life you say you want.

Here is how to use this book:

1. Begin with day one.

2. Do every day in order.

3. Follow the instructions and do them exactly as they are written.

4. Read the Zero Pain Now book through chapter 6. Then stop reading until you reach day 6 in this workbook. If you have already competed the ZPN book that's fine. You can start again. Since understanding is paramount to your long-term success, rereading the book is beneficial.

5. On day 6 complete the Banish Your Pain section in the ZPN book. You can compete the book at your leisure. Make sure to complete the entire book. After completing the Banish Your Pain exercise continue doing all the daily exercises in this workbook. It is doing all the exercises each day that will help you become free of pain and stay free of pain.

Thank you for using the *Zero Pain Now* process.

We want to hear from you. Please send your success stories to: success@zeropainnow.com

Thanks for including me in your journey - Adam

BODY PAIN AUDIT

Use this diagram to identify areas of body pain throughout your life. Use the pages attached to describe the pain, when and how it started, the resolution, and any life events or circumstances happening all that time.

Headache

Upper Back

Mid Back

Lower Back

Sciatic

Thigh

Heel

Foot

Neck

Shoulder

Elbow

Stomach

Wrist

Fingers

Knee

Calf

Ankle

Upper Foot

ADAM HELLER'S

ZERO PAIN NOW

PAIN DESCRIPTION: .... YEAR: ....

HOW STARTED: ....

DIAGNOSIS: ....

SITUATION: ....

....

RESOLUTION: ....

DID PAIN RETURN?: ....

PAIN DESCRIPTION: .... YEAR: ....

HOW STARTED: ....

DIAGNOSIS: ....

SITUATION: ....

....

RESOLUTION: ....

DID PAIN RETURN?: ....

PAIN DESCRIPTION: .... YEAR: ....

HOW STARTED: ....

DIAGNOSIS: ....

SITUATION: ....

....

RESOLUTION: ....

DID PAIN RETURN?: ....

ZERO PAIN NOW

PAIN DESCRIPTION: .... YEAR: ....

HOW STARTED: ....

DIAGNOSIS: ....

SITUATION: ....

....

RESOLUTION: ....

DID PAIN RETURN?: ....

PAIN DESCRIPTION: .... YEAR: ....

HOW STARTED: ....

DIAGNOSIS: ....

SITUATION: ....

....

RESOLUTION: ....

DID PAIN RETURN?: ....

PAIN DESCRIPTION: .... YEAR: ....

HOW STARTED: ....

DIAGNOSIS: ....

SITUATION: ....

....

RESOLUTION: ....

DID PAIN RETURN?: ....

PAIN DESCRIPTION: .... YEAR: ....

HOW STARTED: ....

DIAGNOSIS: ....

SITUATION: ....

....

RESOLUTION: ....

DID PAIN RETURN?: ....

PAIN DESCRIPTION: .... YEAR: ....

HOW STARTED: ....

DIAGNOSIS: ....

SITUATION: ....

....

RESOLUTION: ....

DID PAIN RETURN?: ....

PAIN DESCRIPTION: .... YEAR: ....

HOW STARTED: ....

DIAGNOSIS: ....

SITUATION: ....

....

RESOLUTION: ....

DID PAIN RETURN?: ....

PAIN DESCRIPTION: .... YEAR: ....

HOW STARTED: ....

DIAGNOSIS: ....

SITUATION: ....

....

RESOLUTION: ....

DID PAIN RETURN?: ....

PAIN DESCRIPTION: .... YEAR: ....

HOW STARTED: ....

DIAGNOSIS: ....

SITUATION: ....

....

RESOLUTION: ....

DID PAIN RETURN?: ....

PAIN DESCRIPTION: .... YEAR: ....

HOW STARTED: ....

DIAGNOSIS: ....

SITUATION: ....

....

RESOLUTION: ....

DID PAIN RETURN?: ....

As you perform all the exercises throughout your Zero Pain Now Workbook, notice any changes in your level or location of discomfort.

DAY 1

Today we have a special bonus for you. Adam has created a free video only for people using this workbook to help you optimize your results. If possible please go watch the video before you proceed. The video is available at **http://www.zeropainnow.com/videoday1**

Make a detailed list of everything in your life that is currently producing stress, tension, anger, rage or any other negative emotions. The events may have occurred decades ago or yesterday. The important thing is that they are causing emotions now. Include everything. When you think you are done look and find more.

_____

_____

_____

_____

_____

_____

_____

_____

_____

_____

Spend at least 15 minutes writing about the list you just made. Write everything that enters your mind. Don't censor yourself. Punctuation and spelling are unimportant. Just write as fast as you can. Focus on your emotions. What are they? How do you feel?

_____

_____

_____

_____

_____

_____

_____

_____

_____

_____

_____

_____

_____

_____

_____

_____

_____

_____

_____

_____

_____

_____

_____

_____

_____

_____

_____

_____

Send an e-mail to _workbook@zeropainnow.com_ confirming you performed your tasks along with any updates about your progress. This will help you stay accountable for your daily actions. Also, some of the entries are reviewed by Adam and other trained _Zero Pain Now_ staff who may reply to you with valuable feedback.

DAY 2

Make another detailed list of everything in your life that is currently producing stress, tension, anger, rage, or any negative emotions. The events may have occurred decades ago or yesterday. The important thing is that they are causing emotions now. Include everything. When you think you are done look and find more. Notice if you discovered new items since you made your list yesterday.

_____

_____

_____

_____

_____

_____

_____

_____

_____

_____

_____

_____

_____

_____

Spend at least 15 minutes writing about the list you just made. Write everything that enters your mind. Don't censor yourself. Punctuation and spelling are unimportant. Just write as fast as you can. Focus on your emotions. What are they? How do you feel?

_____

_____

_____

_____

_____

_____

_____

_____

_____

_____

_____

_____

_____

_____

_____

_____

_____

_____

_____

_____

_____

_____

_____

_____

_____

_____

_____

_____

_____

_____

_____

Send an e-mail to *workbook@zeropainnow.com* confirming you performed your tasks along with any updates about your progress. This will help you stay accountable for your daily actions. Also, some of the entries are reviewed by Adam and other trained *Zero Pain Now* staff who may reply to you with valuable feedback.

DAY 3

Make another detailed list of everything in your life that is currently producing stress, tension or negative emotions. The events may have occurred decades ago or yesterday. The important thing is that they are causing emotions now. Include everything. When you think you are done look and find more. Notice if you discovered new items since you made your list yesterday.

_____

_____

_____

_____

_____

_____

_____

_____

_____

_____

_____

_____

_____

_____

Spend at least 15 minutes writing about the list you just made. Write everything that enters your mind. Don't censor yourself. Punctuation and spelling are unimportant. Just write as fast as you can. Focus on your emotions. What are they? How do you feel?

_____

_____

_____

_____

_____

_____

_____

_____

_____

_____

_____

_____

_____

_____

_____

_____

What connection is there between your emotions and your discomfort? Continue to notice the connection. The more you understand the connection the faster you will heal yourself.

_____

_____

_____

_____

_____

_____

_____

_____

_____

_____

_____

_____

Send an e-mail to _workbook@zeropainnow.com_ confirming you performed your tasks along with any updates about your progress. This will help you stay accountable for your daily actions. Also, some of the entries are reviewed by Adam and other trained _Zero Pain Now_ staff who may reply to you with valuable feedback.

DAY 4

Today we have another special extra bonus for you. There is a free video only available to people using this workbook that will help you accelerate your results. If possible go and watch the video before you proceed with the tasks for today. If it isn't possible to watch the video now you can watch at your convenience. The video is available at **http://www.zeropainnow.com/videoday4**

What have you noticed the last few days about the link between your emotions and your symptoms?

_____

_____

_____

_____

_____

_____

_____

_____

_____

_____

_____

_____

What changes (if any) did you notice in your level or location of discomfort while watching the video?

_____

_____

_____

_____

_____

_____

_____

_____

_____

_____

_____

_____

_____

_____

Spend at least 15 minutes writing about the list you just made. Write everything that enters your mind.

Don't censor yourself. Punctuation and spelling are unimportant. Just write as fast as you can. Focus on your

emotions. What are they? How do you feel?

_____

_____

_____

_____

_____

_____

_____

_____

_____

_____

_____

_____

_____

_____

_____

_____

One of the imperative parts of your *Zero Pain Now* healing will be to resume normal physical activity as soon as you believe you can. What physical activities did you do today? What will you commit to do tomorrow? What do you need to tell yourself to banish fear?

_____

_____

_____

_____

_____

_____

_____

_____

_____

_____

_____

_____

_____

Send an e-mail to *workbook@zeropainnow.com* confirming you performed your tasks along with any updates about your progress. This will help you stay accountable for your daily actions. Also, some of the entries are reviewed by Adam and other trained *Zero Pain Now* staff who may reply to you with valuable feedback.

DAY 5

List everything about your career, family relationships, outside relationships and health that add tension, rage or other negative emotions in your life.

_____

_____

_____

_____

_____

_____

_____

_____

_____

_____

_____

_____

_____

_____

_____

_____

_____

_____

What is the connection between these emotions and your discomfort?

_____

_____

_____

_____

_____

_____

How did your family, caretakers or mentors deal with anger and rage? How has your way of dealing with these emotions been affected by them? How could this contribute to your discomfort?

_____

_____

_____

_____

_____

_____

_____

_____

What physical activities did you participate in today?

_____

_____

_____

_____

_____

_____

_____

_____

_____

_____

_____

_____

_____

Send an e-mail to _workbook@zeropainnow.com_ confirming you performed your tasks along with any updates about your progress. This will help you stay accountable for your daily actions. Also, some of the entries are reviewed by Adam and other trained _Zero Pain Now_ staff who may reply to you with valuable feedback.

PATH TO PAIN

Psycho-Physical Activity

Unbearable Emotions
Buried in Unconscious Mind

Change in Autonomic
Nervous System

Reduction of Blood Flow

Oxygen Deprivation
at Effected Location

RESULT

- Muscle Pain
- Nerve Pain
- Tendon Pain
- Numbness
- Tingling
- Weakness

DPS

As you will soon learn and understand, Diversion Pain Syndrome ("DPS") is a psycho-physical activity that produces symptoms including pain, tingling, burning, numbness and weakness.

The process that leads to your pain begins in your brain with repressed emotions. That's why you probably notice that your pain appears or escalates in times of stress or tension. The purpose of DPS is to divert your attention from these repressed emotions to something physical, in your case pain or other symptoms.

As you use the *Zero Pain Now* process to heal your pain you will be identifying the negative emotions that cause and exacerbate your symptoms. The following list will be extremely helpful when you are using the process to heal your pain. The more familiar you are with this list of negative emotions, the easier it will be for you to expedite your becoming pain free.

You can accelerate the process by reading each individual emotion out loud and asking yourself where and when in my life do I feel – name the emotion? The more time you spend checking in with your emotions the more quickly you will be able to permanently heal your pain using the *Zero Pain Now* process.

AFRAID
apprehensive
dread
foreboding
frightened
mistrustful
panicked
scared
suspicious
terrified
Wary
worried

ANNOYED
aggravated
dismayed
disgruntled
displeased
exasperated
frustrated
impatient
irritated
irked

ANGRY
enraged
furious
incensed
indignant
irate
livid
outraged
resentful

AVERSION
animosity
appalled
contempt
disgusted
dislike
hate
horrified
hostile
repulsed

CONFUSED
ambivalent
baffled
bewildered
dazed
hesitant
lost
mystified
perplexed
puzzled
torn

DISCONNECTED
alienated
aloof
apathetic
bored
cold
detached
distant
distracted
indifferent
numb
removed
uninterested
withdrawn

DISQUIET
agitated
alarmed
discombobulated
disconcerted
disturbed
perturbed
rattled
restless
shocked
startled
surprised
troubled
turbulent
turmoil
uncomfortable
uneasy
unnerved
unsettled
upset

EMBARRASSED
ashamed
chagrined
flustered
guilty
mortified
self-conscious

FATIGUE
beat
burnt out
depleted
exhausted
lethargic
listless
sleepy
tired
weary
worn out

PAIN
agony
anguished
bereaved
devastated
grief
heartbroken
hurt
lonely
miserable
regretful
remorseful

SAD
depressed
dejected
despair
despondent
disappointed
discouraged
disheartened
forlorn
gloomy
heavy hearted
hopeless
melancholy
unhappy
wretched

TENSE
anxious
cranky
distressed
distraught
edgy
fidgety
frazzled
irritable
jittery
nervous
overwhelmed
restless
stressed out

VULNERABLE
fragile
guarded
helpless
insecure
leery
reserved
sensitive
shaky

YEARNING
envious
jealous
longing
nostalgic
pining
wistful

©2005 by Center for Nonviolent Communication www.cnvc.org Email: cnvc@cnvc.org Used with Permission

DAY 6

You did your Zero Pain Now Banish Your Pain process today. Now you understand that the real cause of your pain is repressed emotions that don't fit inside your self-image. You learned all about Diversion Pain Syndrome (DPS.) You understand DPS has a purpose. The purpose is to divert your attention from "unbearable" emotions to something physical like pain. Whether you completely or partially banished your pain today is unimportant. What is important is that by changing the way you think, you changed your level of discomfort. This is your proof that the cause could not be structural. The cause must originate in your brain and you are now in control. You can now complete your Zero Pain Now process by finishing becoming and staying pain-free, or if you are now free of pain, staying that way as you resume all normal physical activities and make your new way of thinking about your emotions permanent. Be vigilant. Keep following your plan and do every tasks every day.

Any time you feel any pain immediately stop and ask yourself, "Right Now, what emotion am I feeling?" Answer out loud, "I am feeling _____." Continue until your pain is gone.

Today spend at least 15 consecutive minutes asking yourself the following question: "Right Now, what emotion am I feeling?" Always answer out loud "I am feeling _____."

Spend at least 15 minutes writing about your new strategy for thinking psychologically and everything you discovered today about your emotions.

_____

_____

_____

_____

_____

_____

_____

_____

_____

_____

_____

_____

_____

_____

_____

_____

_____

_____

_____

_____

_____

_____

Send an e-mail to _workbook@zeropainnow.com_ confirming you performed your tasks along with any updates about your progress. This will help you stay accountable for your daily actions. Also, some of the entries are reviewed by Adam and other trained _Zero Pain Now_ staff who may reply to you with valuable feedback.

Look for what has changed. What is better? What can you do that you could not do before?

_____

_____

_____

_____

_____

_____

_____

_____

_____

_____

_____

_____

_____

_____

_____

_____

_____

_____

Spend at least 15 consecutive minutes asking yourself the following question:

"Right Now, what emotion am I feeling?" Always answer out loud and write your answers in the allotted space
"I am feeling _____."

"Right Now, what emotion am I feeling?" Always answer out loud and write your answers in the allotted space
"I am feeling _____."

"Right Now, what emotion am I feeling?" Always answer out loud and write your answers in the allotted space
"I am feeling _____."

"Right Now, what emotion am I feeling?" Always answer out loud and write your answers in the allotted space
"I am feeling _____."

"Right Now, what emotion am I feeling?" Always answer out loud and write your answers in the allotted space
"I am feeling _____."

"Right Now, what emotion am I feeling?" Always answer out loud and write your answers in the allotted space
"I am feeling _____."

"Right Now, what emotion am I feeling?" Always answer out loud and write your answers in the allotted space
"I am feeling _____."

"Right Now, what emotion am I feeling?" Always answer out loud and write your answers in the allotted space
"I am feeling _____."

"Right Now, what emotion am I feeling?" Always answer out loud and write your answers in the allotted space
"I am feeling _____."

"Right Now, what emotion am I feeling?" Always answer out loud and write your answers in the allotted space
"I am feeling _____."

"Right Now, what emotion am I feeling?" Always answer out loud and write your answers in the allotted space
"I am feeling _____."

"Right Now, what emotion am I feeling?" Always answer out loud and write your answers in the allotted space
"I am feeling _____."

"Right Now, what emotion am I feeling?" Always answer out loud and write your answers in the allotted space
"I am feeling _____."

"Right Now, what emotion am I feeling?" Always answer out loud and write your answers in the allotted space
"I am feeling _____."

"Right Now, what emotion am I feeling?" Always answer out loud and write your answers in the allotted space
"I am feeling _____."

"Right Now, what emotion am I feeling?" Always answer out loud and write your answers in the allotted space
"I am feeling _____."

"Right Now, what emotion am I feeling?" Always answer out loud and write your answers in the allotted space
"I am feeling _____."

"Right Now, what emotion am I feeling?" Always answer out loud and write your answers in the allotted space
"I am feeling _____."

"Right Now, what emotion am I feeling?" Always answer out loud and write your answers in the allotted space
"I am feeling _____."

"Right Now, what emotion am I feeling?" Always answer out loud and write your answers in the allotted space
"I am feeling _____."

"Right Now, what emotion am I feeling?" Always answer out loud and write your answers in the allotted space
"I am feeling _____."

"Right Now, what emotion am I feeling?" Always answer out loud and write your answers in the allotted space
"I am feeling _____."

"Right Now, what emotion am I feeling?" Always answer out loud and write your answers in the allotted space
"I am feeling _____."

"Right Now, what emotion am I feeling?" Always answer out loud and write your answers in the allotted space
"I am feeling _____."

Spend at least 10 minutes writing about anything in your life that is producing tension, anger, rage or any negative emotion.

_____

_____

_____

_____

_____

_____

_____

_____

_____

_____

_____

_____

_____

_____

_____

_____

What physical activities did you participate in today?

_____

_____

_____

_____

_____

_____

_____

_____

_____

_____

_____

_____

Send an e-mail to *workbook@zeropainnow.com* confirming you performed your tasks along with any updates about your progress. This will help you stay accountable for your daily actions. Also, some of the entries are reviewed by Adam and other trained *Zero Pain Now* staff who may reply to you with valuable feedback.

DAY 8

Continue to look for what has changed for the better.

Spend at least 15 consecutive minutes asking yourself the following question:

"Right Now, what emotion am I feeling?" Always answer out loud and write your answers in the allotted space "I am feeling _____."

"Right Now, what emotion am I feeling?" Always answer out loud and write your answers in the allotted space "I am feeling _____."

"Right Now, what emotion am I feeling?" Always answer out loud and write your answers in the allotted space "I am feeling _____."

"Right Now, what emotion am I feeling?" Always answer out loud and write your answers in the allotted space "I am feeling _____."

"Right Now, what emotion am I feeling?" Always answer out loud and write your answers in the allotted space "I am feeling _____."

"Right Now, what emotion am I feeling?" Always answer out loud and write your answers in the allotted space "I am feeling _____."

"Right Now, what emotion am I feeling?" Always answer out loud and write your answers in the allotted space "I am feeling _____."

"Right Now, what emotion am I feeling?" Always answer out loud and write your answers in the allotted space "I am feeling _____."

"Right Now, what emotion am I feeling?" Always answer out loud and write your answers in the allotted space "I am feeling _____."

"Right Now, what emotion am I feeling?" Always answer out loud and write your answers in the allotted space "I am feeling _____."

"Right Now, what emotion am I feeling?" Always answer out loud and write your answers in the allotted space "I am feeling _____."

"Right Now, what emotion am I feeling?" Always answer out loud and write your answers in the allotted space "I am feeling _____."

"Right Now, what emotion am I feeling?" Always answer out loud and write your answers in the allotted space
"I am feeling _____."

"Right Now, what emotion am I feeling?" Always answer out loud and write your answers in the allotted space
"I am feeling _____."

"Right Now, what emotion am I feeling?" Always answer out loud and write your answers in the allotted space
"I am feeling _____."

"Right Now, what emotion am I feeling?" Always answer out loud and write your answers in the allotted space
"I am feeling _____."

"Right Now, what emotion am I feeling?" Always answer out loud and write your answers in the allotted space
"I am feeling _____."

"Right Now, what emotion am I feeling?" Always answer out loud and write your answers in the allotted space
"I am feeling _____."

"Right Now, what emotion am I feeling?" Always answer out loud and write your answers in the allotted space
"I am feeling _____."

"Right Now, what emotion am I feeling?" Always answer out loud and write your answers in the allotted space
"I am feeling _____."

"Right Now, what emotion am I feeling?" Always answer out loud and write your answers in the allotted space
"I am feeling _____."

"Right Now, what emotion am I feeling?" Always answer out loud and write your answers in the allotted space
"I am feeling _____."

"Right Now, what emotion am I feeling?" Always answer out loud and write your answers in the allotted space
"I am feeling _____."

"Right Now, what emotion am I feeling?" Always answer out loud and write your answers in the allotted space
"I am feeling _____."

What response are you getting from those around you?

_____

_____

_____

_____

_____

_____

_____

What emotions do you feel about their response?

_____

_____

_____

_____

_____

_____

_____

_____

Were you physically active today? What specifically did you do? Resuming physical activities is paramount to your long-term success.

_____

_____

_____

_____

_____

_____

_____

_____

_____

_____

_____

_____

_____

Send an e-mail to *workbook@zeropainnow.com* confirming you performed your tasks along with any updates about your progress. This will help you stay accountable for your daily actions. Also, some of the entries are reviewed by Adam and other trained *Zero Pain Now* staff who may reply to you with valuable feedback.

DAY 9

Spend at least 15 consecutive minutes asking yourself the following question:

"Right Now, what emotion am I feeling?" Always answer out loud and write your answers in the allotted space
"I am feeling _____."

"Right Now, what emotion am I feeling?" Always answer out loud and write your answers in the allotted space
"I am feeling _____."

"Right Now, what emotion am I feeling?" Always answer out loud and write your answers in the allotted space
"I am feeling _____."

"Right Now, what emotion am I feeling?" Always answer out loud and write your answers in the allotted space
"I am feeling _____."

"Right Now, what emotion am I feeling?" Always answer out loud and write your answers in the allotted space
"I am feeling _____."

"Right Now, what emotion am I feeling?" Always answer out loud and write your answers in the allotted space
"I am feeling _____."

"Right Now, what emotion am I feeling?" Always answer out loud and write your answers in the allotted space
"I am feeling _____."

"Right Now, what emotion am I feeling?" Always answer out loud and write your answers in the allotted space
"I am feeling _____."

"Right Now, what emotion am I feeling?" Always answer out loud and write your answers in the allotted space
"I am feeling _____."

"Right Now, what emotion am I feeling?" Always answer out loud and write your answers in the allotted space
"I am feeling _____."

"Right Now, what emotion am I feeling?" Always answer out loud and write your answers in the allotted space
"I am feeling _____."

"Right Now, what emotion am I feeling?" Always answer out loud and write your answers in the allotted space
"I am feeling _____."

"Right Now, what emotion am I feeling?" Always answer out loud and write your answers in the allotted space
"I am feeling _____."

"Right Now, what emotion am I feeling?" Always answer out loud and write your answers in the allotted space
"I am feeling _____."

"Right Now, what emotion am I feeling?" Always answer out loud and write your answers in the allotted space
"I am feeling _____."

"Right Now, what emotion am I feeling?" Always answer out loud and write your answers in the allotted space
"I am feeling _____."

"Right Now, what emotion am I feeling?" Always answer out loud and write your answers in the allotted space
"I am feeling _____."

"Right Now, what emotion am I feeling?" Always answer out loud and write your answers in the allotted space
"I am feeling _____."

"Right Now, what emotion am I feeling?" Always answer out loud and write your answers in the allotted space
"I am feeling _____."

"Right Now, what emotion am I feeling?" Always answer out loud and write your answers in the allotted space
"I am feeling _____."

"Right Now, what emotion am I feeling?" Always answer out loud and write your answers in the allotted space
"I am feeling _____."

"Right Now, what emotion am I feeling?" Always answer out loud and write your answers in the allotted space
"I am feeling _____."

"Right Now, what emotion am I feeling?" Always answer out loud and write your answers in the allotted space
"I am feeling _____."

"Right Now, what emotion am I feeling?" Always answer out loud and write your answers in the allotted space
"I am feeling _____."

"Right Now, what emotion am I feeling?" Always answer out loud and write your answers in the allotted space
"I am feeling _____."

What is different about the way you manage your emotions?

_____

_____

_____

_____

_____

_____

_____

Are you becoming more active? How specifically?

_____

_____

_____

_____

_____

_____

_____

_____

What did you do today that you were unable to do before?

_____

_____

_____

_____

_____

_____

_____

_____

_____

_____

_____

_____

_____

_____

Send an e-mail to *workbook@zeropainnow.com* confirming you performed your tasks along with any updates about your progress. This will help you stay accountable for your daily actions. Also, some of the entries are reviewed by Adam and other trained *Zero Pain Now* staff who may reply to you with valuable feedback.

DAY 10

Spend at least 15 consecutive minutes asking yourself the following question:

"Right Now, what emotion am I feeling?" Always answer out loud and write your answers in the allotted space
"I am feeling _____."

"Right Now, what emotion am I feeling?" Always answer out loud and write your answers in the allotted space
"I am feeling _____."

"Right Now, what emotion am I feeling?" Always answer out loud and write your answers in the allotted space
"I am feeling _____."

"Right Now, what emotion am I feeling?" Always answer out loud and write your answers in the allotted space
"I am feeling _____."

"Right Now, what emotion am I feeling?" Always answer out loud and write your answers in the allotted space
"I am feeling _____."

"Right Now, what emotion am I feeling?" Always answer out loud and write your answers in the allotted space
"I am feeling _____."

"Right Now, what emotion am I feeling?" Always answer out loud and write your answers in the allotted space
"I am feeling _____."

"Right Now, what emotion am I feeling?" Always answer out loud and write your answers in the allotted space
"I am feeling _____."

"Right Now, what emotion am I feeling?" Always answer out loud and write your answers in the allotted space
"I am feeling _____."

"Right Now, what emotion am I feeling?" Always answer out loud and write your answers in the allotted space
"I am feeling _____."

"Right Now, what emotion am I feeling?" Always answer out loud and write your answers in the allotted space
"I am feeling _____."

"Right Now, what emotion am I feeling?" Always answer out loud and write your answers in the allotted space
"I am feeling _____."

"Right Now, what emotion am I feeling?" Always answer out loud and write your answers in the allotted space
"I am feeling _____."

"Right Now, what emotion am I feeling?" Always answer out loud and write your answers in the allotted space
"I am feeling _____."

"Right Now, what emotion am I feeling?" Always answer out loud and write your answers in the allotted space
"I am feeling _____."

"Right Now, what emotion am I feeling?" Always answer out loud and write your answers in the allotted space
"I am feeling _____."

"Right Now, what emotion am I feeling?" Always answer out loud and write your answers in the allotted space
"I am feeling _____."

"Right Now, what emotion am I feeling?" Always answer out loud and write your answers in the allotted space
"I am feeling _____."

"Right Now, what emotion am I feeling?" Always answer out loud and write your answers in the allotted space
"I am feeling _____."

"Right Now, what emotion am I feeling?" Always answer out loud and write your answers in the allotted space
"I am feeling _____."

"Right Now, what emotion am I feeling?" Always answer out loud and write your answers in the allotted space
"I am feeling _____."

"Right Now, what emotion am I feeling?" Always answer out loud and write your answers in the allotted space
"I am feeling _____."

"Right Now, what emotion am I feeling?" Always answer out loud and write your answers in the allotted space
"I am feeling _____."

"Right Now, what emotion am I feeling?" Always answer out loud and write your answers in the allotted space
"I am feeling _____."

"Right Now, what emotion am I feeling?" Always answer out loud and write your answers in the allotted space
"I am feeling _____."

What's going on in your life? Write for at least 10 minutes.

_____

_____

_____

_____

_____

_____

_____

_____

_____

_____

_____

_____

_____

Send an e-mail to _workbook@zeropainnow.com_ confirming you performed your tasks along with any updates about your progress. This will help you stay accountable for your daily actions. Also, some of the entries are reviewed by Adam and other trained _Zero Pain Now_ staff who may reply to you with valuable feedback.

DAY 11

Clients, including those most successful in responding to the Zero Pain Now process, sometimes go through periods of doubt. Any doubt is the unconscious mind's desire to return to the old method of diversion. Learning your process to ostracize your doubt is an important part of your process.

What (if anything) do you need to do in your brain to be absolutely certain that you have DPS and know that you can control your brain and live free of pain?

_____

_____

_____

_____

_____

_____

_____

_____

_____

_____

_____

_____

_____

_____

Spend at least 15 consecutive minutes asking yourself the following question:

"Right Now, what emotion am I feeling?" Always answer out loud and write your answers in the allotted space
"I am feeling _____."

"Right Now, what emotion am I feeling?" Always answer out loud and write your answers in the allotted space
"I am feeling _____."

"Right Now, what emotion am I feeling?" Always answer out loud and write your answers in the allotted space
"I am feeling _____."

"Right Now, what emotion am I feeling?" Always answer out loud and write your answers in the allotted space
"I am feeling _____."

"Right Now, what emotion am I feeling?" Always answer out loud and write your answers in the allotted space
"I am feeling _____."

"Right Now, what emotion am I feeling?" Always answer out loud and write your answers in the allotted space
"I am feeling _____."

"Right Now, what emotion am I feeling?" Always answer out loud and write your answers in the allotted space
"I am feeling _____."

"Right Now, what emotion am I feeling?" Always answer out loud and write your answers in the allotted space
"I am feeling _____."

"Right Now, what emotion am I feeling?" Always answer out loud and write your answers in the allotted space
"I am feeling _____."

"Right Now, what emotion am I feeling?" Always answer out loud and write your answers in the allotted space
"I am feeling _____."

"Right Now, what emotion am I feeling?" Always answer out loud and write your answers in the allotted space
"I am feeling _____."

"Right Now, what emotion am I feeling?" Always answer out loud and write your answers in the allotted space
"I am feeling _____."

"Right Now, what emotion am I feeling?" Always answer out loud and write your answers in the allotted space
"I am feeling _____."

"Right Now, what emotion am I feeling?" Always answer out loud and write your answers in the allotted space
"I am feeling _____."

"Right Now, what emotion am I feeling?" Always answer out loud and write your answers in the allotted space
"I am feeling _____."

"Right Now, what emotion am I feeling?" Always answer out loud and write your answers in the allotted space
"I am feeling _____."

"Right Now, what emotion am I feeling?" Always answer out loud and write your answers in the allotted space
"I am feeling _____."

"Right Now, what emotion am I feeling?" Always answer out loud and write your answers in the allotted space
"I am feeling _____."

"Right Now, what emotion am I feeling?" Always answer out loud and write your answers in the allotted space
"I am feeling _____."

"Right Now, what emotion am I feeling?" Always answer out loud and write your answers in the allotted space
"I am feeling _____."

"Right Now, what emotion am I feeling?" Always answer out loud and write your answers in the allotted space
"I am feeling _____."

"Right Now, what emotion am I feeling?" Always answer out loud and write your answers in the allotted space
"I am feeling _____."

"Right Now, what emotion am I feeling?" Always answer out loud and write your answers in the allotted space
"I am feeling _____."

"Right Now, what emotion am I feeling?" Always answer out loud and write your answers in the allotted space
"I am feeling _____."

Did you participate in physical activities today? What did you do? What is something more physical that you are ready to do tomorrow?

_____

_____

_____

_____

_____

_____

_____

_____

_____

_____

_____

_____

Send an e-mail to *workbook@zeropainnow.com* confirming you performed your tasks along with any updates about your progress. This will help you stay accountable for your daily actions. Also, some of the entries are reviewed by Adam and other trained *Zero Pain Now* staff who may reply to you with valuable feedback.

DAY 12

How are you now responding differently to situations? Personal relationships? Career? Family?

_____

_____

_____

_____

_____

_____

_____

What is possible for you now that was not possible before?

_____

_____

_____

_____

_____

_____

_____

_____

Are you finding that you are automatically thinking psychologically and noticing your emotions?

_____

_____

_____

_____

_____

_____

What did you do that was physical today? What are you noticing has changed?

_____

_____

_____

_____

_____

_____

Send an e-mail to _workbook@zeropainnow.com_ confirming you performed your tasks along with any updates about your progress. This will help you stay accountable for your daily actions. Also, some of the entries are reviewed by Adam and other trained _Zero Pain Now_ staff who may reply to you with valuable feedback.

What were the 3 events in your life when you were most angry? How do you now feel about those events?

_____

_____

_____

_____

_____

_____

_____

_____

_____

_____

_____

_____

_____

_____

_____

_____

_____

_____

Spend at least 15 consecutive minutes asking yourself the following question:

"Right Now, what emotion am I feeling?" Always answer out loud and write your answers in the allotted space
"I am feeling _____."

"Right Now, what emotion am I feeling?" Always answer out loud and write your answers in the allotted space
"I am feeling _____."

"Right Now, what emotion am I feeling?" Always answer out loud and write your answers in the allotted space
"I am feeling _____."

"Right Now, what emotion am I feeling?" Always answer out loud and write your answers in the allotted space
"I am feeling _____."

"Right Now, what emotion am I feeling?" Always answer out loud and write your answers in the allotted space
"I am feeling _____."

"Right Now, what emotion am I feeling?" Always answer out loud and write your answers in the allotted space
"I am feeling _____."

"Right Now, what emotion am I feeling?" Always answer out loud and write your answers in the allotted space
"I am feeling _____."

"Right Now, what emotion am I feeling?" Always answer out loud and write your answers in the allotted space
"I am feeling _____."

"Right Now, what emotion am I feeling?" Always answer out loud and write your answers in the allotted space
"I am feeling _____."

"Right Now, what emotion am I feeling?" Always answer out loud and write your answers in the allotted space
"I am feeling _____."

"Right Now, what emotion am I feeling?" Always answer out loud and write your answers in the allotted space
"I am feeling _____."

"Right Now, what emotion am I feeling?" Always answer out loud and write your answers in the allotted space
"I am feeling _____."

"Right Now, what emotion am I feeling?" Always answer out loud and write your answers in the allotted space
"I am feeling _____."

"Right Now, what emotion am I feeling?" Always answer out loud and write your answers in the allotted space
"I am feeling _____."

"Right Now, what emotion am I feeling?" Always answer out loud and write your answers in the allotted space
"I am feeling _____."

"Right Now, what emotion am I feeling?" Always answer out loud and write your answers in the allotted space
"I am feeling _____."

"Right Now, what emotion am I feeling?" Always answer out loud and write your answers in the allotted space
"I am feeling _____."

"Right Now, what emotion am I feeling?" Always answer out loud and write your answers in the allotted space
"I am feeling _____."

"Right Now, what emotion am I feeling?" Always answer out loud and write your answers in the allotted space
"I am feeling _____."

"Right Now, what emotion am I feeling?" Always answer out loud and write your answers in the allotted space
"I am feeling _____."

"Right Now, what emotion am I feeling?" Always answer out loud and write your answers in the allotted space
"I am feeling _____."

"Right Now, what emotion am I feeling?" Always answer out loud and write your answers in the allotted space
"I am feeling _____."

"Right Now, what emotion am I feeling?" Always answer out loud and write your answers in the allotted space
"I am feeling _____."

Send an e-mail to *workbook@zeropainnow.com* confirming you performed your tasks along with any updates about your progress. This will help you stay accountable for your daily actions. Also, some of the entries are reviewed by Adam and other trained *Zero Pain Now* staff who may reply to you with valuable feedback.

DAY 14

One of my favorite quotes is "The cost of freedom is responsibility." What do you now know about your responsibility for your DPS?

What is now different and better in your life? List everything.

_____

_____

_____

_____

_____

Is there anyone or anything in your life that you need to banish? Are you willing to do this for yourself? What emotions do you feel as you ponder this?

_____

_____

_____

_____

_____

_____

_____

Spend at least 15 consecutive minutes asking yourself the following question:

"Right Now, what emotion am I feeling?" Always answer out loud and write your answers in the allotted space
"I am feeling _____."

"Right Now, what emotion am I feeling?" Always answer out loud and write your answers in the allotted space
"I am feeling _____."

"Right Now, what emotion am I feeling?" Always answer out loud and write your answers in the allotted space
"I am feeling _____."

"Right Now, what emotion am I feeling?" Always answer out loud and write your answers in the allotted space
"I am feeling _____."

"Right Now, what emotion am I feeling?" Always answer out loud and write your answers in the allotted space
"I am feeling _____."

"Right Now, what emotion am I feeling?" Always answer out loud and write your answers in the allotted space
"I am feeling _____."

"Right Now, what emotion am I feeling?" Always answer out loud and write your answers in the allotted space
"I am feeling _____."

"Right Now, what emotion am I feeling?" Always answer out loud and write your answers in the allotted space
"I am feeling _____."

"Right Now, what emotion am I feeling?" Always answer out loud and write your answers in the allotted space
"I am feeling _____."

"Right Now, what emotion am I feeling?" Always answer out loud and write your answers in the allotted space
"I am feeling _____."

"Right Now, what emotion am I feeling?" Always answer out loud and write your answers in the allotted space
"I am feeling _____."

"Right Now, what emotion am I feeling?" Always answer out loud and write your answers in the allotted space
"I am feeling _____."

"Right Now, what emotion am I feeling?" Always answer out loud and write your answers in the allotted space
"I am feeling _____."

"Right Now, what emotion am I feeling?" Always answer out loud and write your answers in the allotted space
"I am feeling _____."

"Right Now, what emotion am I feeling?" Always answer out loud and write your answers in the allotted space
"I am feeling _____."

"Right Now, what emotion am I feeling?" Always answer out loud and write your answers in the allotted space
"I am feeling _____."

"Right Now, what emotion am I feeling?" Always answer out loud and write your answers in the allotted space
"I am feeling _____."

"Right Now, what emotion am I feeling?" Always answer out loud and write your answers in the allotted space
"I am feeling _____."

"Right Now, what emotion am I feeling?" Always answer out loud and write your answers in the allotted space
"I am feeling _____."

"Right Now, what emotion am I feeling?" Always answer out loud and write your answers in the allotted space
"I am feeling _____."

"Right Now, what emotion am I feeling?" Always answer out loud and write your answers in the allotted space
"I am feeling _____."

"Right Now, what emotion am I feeling?" Always answer out loud and write your answers in the allotted space
"I am feeling _____."

"Right Now, what emotion am I feeling?" Always answer out loud and write your answers in the allotted space
"I am feeling _____."

Send an e-mail to *workbook@zeropainnow.com* confirming you performed your tasks along with any updates about your progress. This will help you stay accountable for your daily actions. Also, some of the entries are reviewed by Adam and other trained *Zero Pain Now* staff who may reply to you with valuable feedback.

ZERO PAIN NOW

DAY 15

WOW! You have completed 2 weeks. Today is the day for you to celebrate your effort, persistence and dedication to healing yourself.

Choose something you will do for yourself today. Perhaps a movie? Massage? Long walk in the country? Some enjoyable physical activity that you have been unable to do? Choose something to thank yourself and do it.

Send an e-mail to *workbook@zeropainnow.com* confirming you performed your tasks along with any updates about your progress. This will help you stay accountable for your daily actions. Also, some of the entries are reviewed by Adam and other trained *Zero Pain Now* staff who may reply to you with valuable feedback.

DAY 16

Where have you noticed other people repressing emotions and causing themselves to suffer?

_____

_____

_____

_____

_____

_____

_____

_____

_____

_____

_____

_____

_____

_____

_____

_____

_____

Spend at least 15 consecutive minutes asking yourself the following question:

"Right Now, what emotion am I feeling?" Always answer out loud and write your answers in the allotted space
"I am feeling _____."

"Right Now, what emotion am I feeling?" Always answer out loud and write your answers in the allotted space
"I am feeling _____."

"Right Now, what emotion am I feeling?" Always answer out loud and write your answers in the allotted space
"I am feeling _____."

"Right Now, what emotion am I feeling?" Always answer out loud and write your answers in the allotted space
"I am feeling _____."

"Right Now, what emotion am I feeling?" Always answer out loud and write your answers in the allotted space
"I am feeling _____."

"Right Now, what emotion am I feeling?" Always answer out loud and write your answers in the allotted space
"I am feeling _____."

"Right Now, what emotion am I feeling?" Always answer out loud and write your answers in the allotted space
"I am feeling _____."

"Right Now, what emotion am I feeling?" Always answer out loud and write your answers in the allotted space
"I am feeling _____."

"Right Now, what emotion am I feeling?" Always answer out loud and write your answers in the allotted space
"I am feeling _____."

"Right Now, what emotion am I feeling?" Always answer out loud and write your answers in the allotted space
"I am feeling _____."

"Right Now, what emotion am I feeling?" Always answer out loud and write your answers in the allotted space
"I am feeling _____."

"Right Now, what emotion am I feeling?" Always answer out loud and write your answers in the allotted space
"I am feeling _____."

"Right Now, what emotion am I feeling?" Always answer out loud and write your answers in the allotted space
"I am feeling _____."

"Right Now, what emotion am I feeling?" Always answer out loud and write your answers in the allotted space
"I am feeling _____."

"Right Now, what emotion am I feeling?" Always answer out loud and write your answers in the allotted space
"I am feeling _____."

"Right Now, what emotion am I feeling?" Always answer out loud and write your answers in the allotted space
"I am feeling _____."

"Right Now, what emotion am I feeling?" Always answer out loud and write your answers in the allotted space
"I am feeling _____."

"Right Now, what emotion am I feeling?" Always answer out loud and write your answers in the allotted space
"I am feeling _____."

"Right Now, what emotion am I feeling?" Always answer out loud and write your answers in the allotted space
"I am feeling _____."

"Right Now, what emotion am I feeling?" Always answer out loud and write your answers in the allotted space
"I am feeling _____."

"Right Now, what emotion am I feeling?" Always answer out loud and write your answers in the allotted space
"I am feeling _____."

"Right Now, what emotion am I feeling?" Always answer out loud and write your answers in the allotted space
"I am feeling _____."

"Right Now, what emotion am I feeling?" Always answer out loud and write your answers in the allotted space
"I am feeling _____."

"Right Now, what emotion am I feeling?" Always answer out loud and write your answers in the allotted space
"I am feeling _____."

"Right Now, what emotion am I feeling?" Always answer out loud and write your answers in the allotted space
"I am feeling _____."

Are you getting more physical? How? What more are you ready to do?

_____

_____

_____

_____

_____

_____

_____

_____

_____

_____

_____

_____

_____

Send an e-mail to *workbook@zeropainnow.com* confirming you performed your tasks along with any updates about your progress. This will help you stay accountable for your daily actions. Also, some of the entries are reviewed by Adam and other trained *Zero Pain Now* staff who may reply to you with valuable feedback.

DAY 17

What events in your life continue to produce tension, anger or rage?

_____

_____

_____

_____

_____

Are you now able to quickly notice your emotions?

_____

_____

_____

_____

_____

Now that you notice your emotions, are you making new and better choices about how you respond?

_____

_____

_____

_____

_____

ZERO PAIN NOW

Spend at least 15 consecutive minutes asking yourself the following question:

"Right Now, what emotion am I feeling?" Always answer out loud and write your answers in the allotted space
"I am feeling _____."

"Right Now, what emotion am I feeling?" Always answer out loud and write your answers in the allotted space
"I am feeling _____."

"Right Now, what emotion am I feeling?" Always answer out loud and write your answers in the allotted space
"I am feeling _____."

"Right Now, what emotion am I feeling?" Always answer out loud and write your answers in the allotted space
"I am feeling _____."

"Right Now, what emotion am I feeling?" Always answer out loud and write your answers in the allotted space
"I am feeling _____."

"Right Now, what emotion am I feeling?" Always answer out loud and write your answers in the allotted space
"I am feeling _____."

"Right Now, what emotion am I feeling?" Always answer out loud and write your answers in the allotted space
"I am feeling _____."

"Right Now, what emotion am I feeling?" Always answer out loud and write your answers in the allotted space
"I am feeling _____."

"Right Now, what emotion am I feeling?" Always answer out loud and write your answers in the allotted space
"I am feeling _____."

"Right Now, what emotion am I feeling?" Always answer out loud and write your answers in the allotted space
"I am feeling _____."

"Right Now, what emotion am I feeling?" Always answer out loud and write your answers in the allotted space
"I am feeling _____."

"Right Now, what emotion am I feeling?" Always answer out loud and write your answers in the allotted space
"I am feeling _____."

"Right Now, what emotion am I feeling?" Always answer out loud and write your answers in the allotted space
"I am feeling _____."

"Right Now, what emotion am I feeling?" Always answer out loud and write your answers in the allotted space
"I am feeling _____."

"Right Now, what emotion am I feeling?" Always answer out loud and write your answers in the allotted space
"I am feeling _____."

"Right Now, what emotion am I feeling?" Always answer out loud and write your answers in the allotted space
"I am feeling _____."

"Right Now, what emotion am I feeling?" Always answer out loud and write your answers in the allotted space
"I am feeling _____."

"Right Now, what emotion am I feeling?" Always answer out loud and write your answers in the allotted space
"I am feeling _____."

"Right Now, what emotion am I feeling?" Always answer out loud and write your answers in the allotted space
"I am feeling _____."

"Right Now, what emotion am I feeling?" Always answer out loud and write your answers in the allotted space
"I am feeling _____."

"Right Now, what emotion am I feeling?" Always answer out loud and write your answers in the allotted space
"I am feeling _____."

"Right Now, what emotion am I feeling?" Always answer out loud and write your answers in the allotted space
"I am feeling _____."

Send an e-mail to *workbook@zeropainnow.com* confirming you performed your tasks along with any updates about your progress. This will help you stay accountable for your daily actions. Also, some of the entries are reviewed by Adam and other trained *Zero Pain Now* staff who may reply to you with valuable feedback.

DAY 18

How do you feel differently about yourself? In what ways is your self-image better?

_____

_____

_____

_____

_____

_____

Did you notice that you are thinking psychologically and noticing what emotions you are feeling?

_____

_____

_____

_____

Even though you do not need to "fix" anything to be free of DPS pain, are there any changes you are willing to make to have a better life?

_____

_____

_____

_____

_____

_____

Spend at least 15 consecutive minutes asking yourself the following question:

"Right Now, what emotion am I feeling?" Always answer out loud and write your answers in the allotted space
"I am feeling _____."

"Right Now, what emotion am I feeling?" Always answer out loud and write your answers in the allotted space
"I am feeling _____."

"Right Now, what emotion am I feeling?" Always answer out loud and write your answers in the allotted space
"I am feeling _____."

"Right Now, what emotion am I feeling?" Always answer out loud and write your answers in the allotted space
"I am feeling _____."

"Right Now, what emotion am I feeling?" Always answer out loud and write your answers in the allotted space
"I am feeling _____."

"Right Now, what emotion am I feeling?" Always answer out loud and write your answers in the allotted space
"I am feeling _____."

"Right Now, what emotion am I feeling?" Always answer out loud and write your answers in the allotted space
"I am feeling _____."

"Right Now, what emotion am I feeling?" Always answer out loud and write your answers in the allotted space
"I am feeling _____."

"Right Now, what emotion am I feeling?" Always answer out loud and write your answers in the allotted space
"I am feeling _____."

"Right Now, what emotion am I feeling?" Always answer out loud and write your answers in the allotted space
"I am feeling _____."

"Right Now, what emotion am I feeling?" Always answer out loud and write your answers in the allotted space
"I am feeling _____."

"Right Now, what emotion am I feeling?" Always answer out loud and write your answers in the allotted space
"I am feeling _____."

"Right Now, what emotion am I feeling?" Always answer out loud and write your answers in the allotted space
"I am feeling _____."

"Right Now, what emotion am I feeling?" Always answer out loud and write your answers in the allotted space
"I am feeling _____."

"Right Now, what emotion am I feeling?" Always answer out loud and write your answers in the allotted space
"I am feeling _____."

"Right Now, what emotion am I feeling?" Always answer out loud and write your answers in the allotted space
"I am feeling _____."

"Right Now, what emotion am I feeling?" Always answer out loud and write your answers in the allotted space
"I am feeling _____."

"Right Now, what emotion am I feeling?" Always answer out loud and write your answers in the allotted space
"I am feeling _____."

"Right Now, what emotion am I feeling?" Always answer out loud and write your answers in the allotted space
"I am feeling _____."

"Right Now, what emotion am I feeling?" Always answer out loud and write your answers in the allotted space
"I am feeling _____."

"Right Now, what emotion am I feeling?" Always answer out loud and write your answers in the allotted space
"I am feeling _____."

"Right Now, what emotion am I feeling?" Always answer out loud and write your answers in the allotted space
"I am feeling _____."

"Right Now, what emotion am I feeling?" Always answer out loud and write your answers in the allotted space
"I am feeling _____."

Send an e-mail to *workbook@zeropainnow.com* confirming you performed your tasks along with any updates about your progress. This will help you stay accountable for your daily actions. Also, some of the entries are reviewed by Adam and other trained *Zero Pain Now* staff who may reply to you with valuable feedback.

DAY 19

Where and when in your life are you too self-critical? What emotions does that behavior produce?

_____

_____

_____

_____

_____

_____

_____

_____

How can you achieve better results and have a gentler more productive self-talk?

_____

_____

_____

_____

_____

_____

_____

Spend at least 15 consecutive minutes asking yourself the following question:

"Right Now, what emotion am I feeling?" Always answer out loud and write your answers in the allotted space
"I am feeling _____."

"Right Now, what emotion am I feeling?" Always answer out loud and write your answers in the allotted space
"I am feeling _____."

"Right Now, what emotion am I feeling?" Always answer out loud and write your answers in the allotted space
"I am feeling _____."

"Right Now, what emotion am I feeling?" Always answer out loud and write your answers in the allotted space
"I am feeling _____."

"Right Now, what emotion am I feeling?" Always answer out loud and write your answers in the allotted space
"I am feeling _____."

"Right Now, what emotion am I feeling?" Always answer out loud and write your answers in the allotted space
"I am feeling _____."

"Right Now, what emotion am I feeling?" Always answer out loud and write your answers in the allotted space
"I am feeling _____."

"Right Now, what emotion am I feeling?" Always answer out loud and write your answers in the allotted space
"I am feeling _____."

"Right Now, what emotion am I feeling?" Always answer out loud and write your answers in the allotted space
"I am feeling _____."

"Right Now, what emotion am I feeling?" Always answer out loud and write your answers in the allotted space
"I am feeling _____."

"Right Now, what emotion am I feeling?" Always answer out loud and write your answers in the allotted space
"I am feeling _____."

"Right Now, what emotion am I feeling?" Always answer out loud and write your answers in the allotted space
"I am feeling _____."

"Right Now, what emotion am I feeling?" Always answer out loud and write your answers in the allotted space

"I am feeling _____."

"Right Now, what emotion am I feeling?" Always answer out loud and write your answers in the allotted space

"I am feeling _____."

"Right Now, what emotion am I feeling?" Always answer out loud and write your answers in the allotted space

"I am feeling _____."

"Right Now, what emotion am I feeling?" Always answer out loud and write your answers in the allotted space

"I am feeling _____."

"Right Now, what emotion am I feeling?" Always answer out loud and write your answers in the allotted space

"I am feeling _____."

"Right Now, what emotion am I feeling?" Always answer out loud and write your answers in the allotted space

"I am feeling _____."

"Right Now, what emotion am I feeling?" Always answer out loud and write your answers in the allotted space

"I am feeling _____."

"Right Now, what emotion am I feeling?" Always answer out loud and write your answers in the allotted space

"I am feeling _____."

"Right Now, what emotion am I feeling?" Always answer out loud and write your answers in the allotted space

"I am feeling _____."

"Right Now, what emotion am I feeling?" Always answer out loud and write your answers in the allotted space

"I am feeling _____."

"Right Now, what emotion am I feeling?" Always answer out loud and write your answers in the allotted space

"I am feeling _____."

Send an e-mail to *workbook@zeropainnow.com* confirming you performed your tasks along with any updates about your progress. This will help you stay accountable for your daily actions. Also, some of the entries are reviewed by Adam and other trained *Zero Pain Now* staff who may reply to you with valuable feedback.

DAY 20

Time to make a new list of everything in your life that produces stress, tension, anger or rage. List everything.

_____

_____

_____

_____

_____

_____

_____

_____

_____

_____

_____

_____

_____

_____

_____

_____

_____

How has your list changed from your earlier lists?

_____

_____

_____

_____

_____

Is there a person or situation that you are ready to remove from your life and your list? Describe.

_____

_____

_____

_____

_____

What emotion do you feel as you think about this?

_____

_____

_____

_____

_____

Spend at least 15 consecutive minutes asking yourself the following question:

"Right Now, what emotion am I feeling?" Always answer out loud and write your answers in the allotted space
"I am feeling _____."

"Right Now, what emotion am I feeling?" Always answer out loud and write your answers in the allotted space
"I am feeling _____."

"Right Now, what emotion am I feeling?" Always answer out loud and write your answers in the allotted space
"I am feeling _____."

"Right Now, what emotion am I feeling?" Always answer out loud and write your answers in the allotted space
"I am feeling _____."

"Right Now, what emotion am I feeling?" Always answer out loud and write your answers in the allotted space
"I am feeling _____."

"Right Now, what emotion am I feeling?" Always answer out loud and write your answers in the allotted space
"I am feeling _____."

"Right Now, what emotion am I feeling?" Always answer out loud and write your answers in the allotted space
"I am feeling _____."

"Right Now, what emotion am I feeling?" Always answer out loud and write your answers in the allotted space
"I am feeling _____."

"Right Now, what emotion am I feeling?" Always answer out loud and write your answers in the allotted space
"I am feeling _____."

"Right Now, what emotion am I feeling?" Always answer out loud and write your answers in the allotted space
"I am feeling _____."

"Right Now, what emotion am I feeling?" Always answer out loud and write your answers in the allotted space
"I am feeling _____."

"Right Now, what emotion am I feeling?" Always answer out loud and write your answers in the allotted space
"I am feeling _____."

"Right Now, what emotion am I feeling?" Always answer out loud and write your answers in the allotted space "I am feeling _____."

"Right Now, what emotion am I feeling?" Always answer out loud and write your answers in the allotted space "I am feeling _____."

"Right Now, what emotion am I feeling?" Always answer out loud and write your answers in the allotted space "I am feeling _____."

"Right Now, what emotion am I feeling?" Always answer out loud and write your answers in the allotted space "I am feeling _____."

"Right Now, what emotion am I feeling?" Always answer out loud and write your answers in the allotted space "I am feeling _____."

"Right Now, what emotion am I feeling?" Always answer out loud and write your answers in the allotted space "I am feeling _____."

"Right Now, what emotion am I feeling?" Always answer out loud and write your answers in the allotted space "I am feeling _____."

"Right Now, what emotion am I feeling?" Always answer out loud and write your answers in the allotted space "I am feeling _____."

"Right Now, what emotion am I feeling?" Always answer out loud and write your answers in the allotted space "I am feeling _____."

"Right Now, what emotion am I feeling?" Always answer out loud and write your answers in the allotted space "I am feeling _____."

"Right Now, what emotion am I feeling?" Always answer out loud and write your answers in the allotted space "I am feeling _____."

Send an e-mail to *workbook@zeropainnow.com* confirming you performed your tasks along with any updates about your progress. This will help you stay accountable for your daily actions. Also, some of the entries are reviewed by Adam and other trained *Zero Pain Now* staff who may reply to you with valuable feedback.

DAY 21

How are you becoming more physically active? What specifically are you doing?

_____

_____

_____

_____

_____

How has your increased physical activity affected the way you feel about yourself?

_____

_____

_____

_____

_____

What are you now noticing about the emotions you are feeling?

_____

_____

_____

_____

Spend at least 15 consecutive minutes asking yourself the following question:

"Right Now, what emotion am I feeling?" Always answer out loud and write your answers in the allotted space
"I am feeling _____."

"Right Now, what emotion am I feeling?" Always answer out loud and write your answers in the allotted space
"I am feeling _____."

"Right Now, what emotion am I feeling?" Always answer out loud and write your answers in the allotted space
"I am feeling _____."

"Right Now, what emotion am I feeling?" Always answer out loud and write your answers in the allotted space
"I am feeling _____."

"Right Now, what emotion am I feeling?" Always answer out loud and write your answers in the allotted space
"I am feeling _____."

"Right Now, what emotion am I feeling?" Always answer out loud and write your answers in the allotted space
"I am feeling _____."

"Right Now, what emotion am I feeling?" Always answer out loud and write your answers in the allotted space
"I am feeling _____."

"Right Now, what emotion am I feeling?" Always answer out loud and write your answers in the allotted space
"I am feeling _____."

"Right Now, what emotion am I feeling?" Always answer out loud and write your answers in the allotted space
"I am feeling _____."

"Right Now, what emotion am I feeling?" Always answer out loud and write your answers in the allotted space
"I am feeling _____."

"Right Now, what emotion am I feeling?" Always answer out loud and write your answers in the allotted space
"I am feeling _____."

"Right Now, what emotion am I feeling?" Always answer out loud and write your answers in the allotted space
"I am feeling _____."

"Right Now, what emotion am I feeling?" Always answer out loud and write your answers in the allotted space
"I am feeling _____."

"Right Now, what emotion am I feeling?" Always answer out loud and write your answers in the allotted space
"I am feeling _____."

"Right Now, what emotion am I feeling?" Always answer out loud and write your answers in the allotted space
"I am feeling _____."

"Right Now, what emotion am I feeling?" Always answer out loud and write your answers in the allotted space
"I am feeling _____."

"Right Now, what emotion am I feeling?" Always answer out loud and write your answers in the allotted space
"I am feeling _____."

"Right Now, what emotion am I feeling?" Always answer out loud and write your answers in the allotted space
"I am feeling _____."

"Right Now, what emotion am I feeling?" Always answer out loud and write your answers in the allotted space
"I am feeling _____."

"Right Now, what emotion am I feeling?" Always answer out loud and write your answers in the allotted space
"I am feeling _____."

"Right Now, what emotion am I feeling?" Always answer out loud and write your answers in the allotted space
"I am feeling _____."

"Right Now, what emotion am I feeling?" Always answer out loud and write your answers in the allotted space
"I am feeling _____."

"Right Now, what emotion am I feeling?" Always answer out loud and write your answers in the allotted space
"I am feeling _____."

Send an e-mail to *workbook@zeropainnow.com* confirming you performed your tasks along with any updates about your progress. This will help you stay accountable for your daily actions. Also, some of the entries are reviewed by Adam and other trained *Zero Pain Now* staff who may reply to you with valuable feedback.

DAY 22

You have completed 3 weeks. Fantastic! Today just notice how you have changed your life.

Send an e-mail to *workbook@zeropainnow.com* confirming you performed your tasks along with any updates about your progress. This will help you stay accountable for your daily actions. Also, some of the entries are reviewed by Adam and other trained *Zero Pain Now* staff who may reply to you with valuable feedback.

DAY 23

How has your default way of thinking about your emotions changed? Are you now automatically paying attention to how you feel about things? Are you noticing and acknowledging when you are angry? Sad? Guilty? Hurt? Ashamed? Are you now thinking psychologically?

_____

_____

_____

_____

_____

_____

_____

_____

_____

_____

_____

_____

_____

_____

_____

_____

_____

Spend at least 15 consecutive minutes asking yourself the following question:

"Right Now, what emotion am I feeling?" Always answer out loud and write your answers in the allotted space
"I am feeling _____."

"Right Now, what emotion am I feeling?" Always answer out loud and write your answers in the allotted space
"I am feeling _____."

"Right Now, what emotion am I feeling?" Always answer out loud and write your answers in the allotted space
"I am feeling _____."

"Right Now, what emotion am I feeling?" Always answer out loud and write your answers in the allotted space
"I am feeling _____."

"Right Now, what emotion am I feeling?" Always answer out loud and write your answers in the allotted space
"I am feeling _____."

"Right Now, what emotion am I feeling?" Always answer out loud and write your answers in the allotted space
"I am feeling _____."

"Right Now, what emotion am I feeling?" Always answer out loud and write your answers in the allotted space
"I am feeling _____."

"Right Now, what emotion am I feeling?" Always answer out loud and write your answers in the allotted space
"I am feeling _____."

"Right Now, what emotion am I feeling?" Always answer out loud and write your answers in the allotted space
"I am feeling _____."

"Right Now, what emotion am I feeling?" Always answer out loud and write your answers in the allotted space
"I am feeling _____."

"Right Now, what emotion am I feeling?" Always answer out loud and write your answers in the allotted space
"I am feeling _____."

"Right Now, what emotion am I feeling?" Always answer out loud and write your answers in the allotted space
"I am feeling _____."

"Right Now, what emotion am I feeling?" Always answer out loud and write your answers in the allotted space
"I am feeling _____."

"Right Now, what emotion am I feeling?" Always answer out loud and write your answers in the allotted space
"I am feeling _____."

"Right Now, what emotion am I feeling?" Always answer out loud and write your answers in the allotted space
"I am feeling _____."

"Right Now, what emotion am I feeling?" Always answer out loud and write your answers in the allotted space
"I am feeling _____."

"Right Now, what emotion am I feeling?" Always answer out loud and write your answers in the allotted space
"I am feeling _____."

"Right Now, what emotion am I feeling?" Always answer out loud and write your answers in the allotted space
"I am feeling _____."

"Right Now, what emotion am I feeling?" Always answer out loud and write your answers in the allotted space
"I am feeling _____."

"Right Now, what emotion am I feeling?" Always answer out loud and write your answers in the allotted space
"I am feeling _____."

"Right Now, what emotion am I feeling?" Always answer out loud and write your answers in the allotted space
"I am feeling _____."

"Right Now, what emotion am I feeling?" Always answer out loud and write your answers in the allotted space
"I am feeling _____."

"Right Now, what emotion am I feeling?" Always answer out loud and write your answers in the allotted space
"I am feeling _____."

"Right Now, what emotion am I feeling?" Always answer out loud and write your answers in the allotted space
"I am feeling _____."

"Right Now, what emotion am I feeling?" Always answer out loud and write your answers in the allotted space
"I am feeling _____."

What did you do today that was physical? What will you do to increase your physical activities?

_____

_____

_____

_____

_____

_____

_____

_____

_____

_____

_____

_____

_____

_____

Send an e-mail to *workbook@zeropainnow.com* confirming you performed your tasks along with any updates about your progress. This will help you stay accountable for your daily actions. Also, some of the entries are reviewed by Adam and other trained *Zero Pain Now* staff who may reply to you with valuable feedback.

ZERO PAIN NOW

DAY 24

Spend at least 15 consecutive minutes asking yourself the following question:

"Right Now, what emotion am I feeling?" Always answer out loud and write your answers in the allotted space
"I am feeling _____."

"Right Now, what emotion am I feeling?" Always answer out loud and write your answers in the allotted space
"I am feeling _____."

"Right Now, what emotion am I feeling?" Always answer out loud and write your answers in the allotted space
"I am feeling _____."

"Right Now, what emotion am I feeling?" Always answer out loud and write your answers in the allotted space
"I am feeling _____."

"Right Now, what emotion am I feeling?" Always answer out loud and write your answers in the allotted space
"I am feeling _____."

"Right Now, what emotion am I feeling?" Always answer out loud and write your answers in the allotted space
"I am feeling _____."

"Right Now, what emotion am I feeling?" Always answer out loud and write your answers in the allotted space
"I am feeling _____."

"Right Now, what emotion am I feeling?" Always answer out loud and write your answers in the allotted space
"I am feeling _____."

"Right Now, what emotion am I feeling?" Always answer out loud and write your answers in the allotted space
"I am feeling _____."

"Right Now, what emotion am I feeling?" Always answer out loud and write your answers in the allotted space
"I am feeling _____."

"Right Now, what emotion am I feeling?" Always answer out loud and write your answers in the allotted space
"I am feeling _____."

"Right Now, what emotion am I feeling?" Always answer out loud and write your answers in the allotted space
"I am feeling _____."

"Right Now, what emotion am I feeling?" Always answer out loud and write your answers in the allotted space
"I am feeling _____."

"Right Now, what emotion am I feeling?" Always answer out loud and write your answers in the allotted space
"I am feeling _____."

"Right Now, what emotion am I feeling?" Always answer out loud and write your answers in the allotted space
"I am feeling _____."

"Right Now, what emotion am I feeling?" Always answer out loud and write your answers in the allotted space
"I am feeling _____."

"Right Now, what emotion am I feeling?" Always answer out loud and write your answers in the allotted space
"I am feeling _____."

"Right Now, what emotion am I feeling?" Always answer out loud and write your answers in the allotted space
"I am feeling _____."

"Right Now, what emotion am I feeling?" Always answer out loud and write your answers in the allotted space
"I am feeling _____."

"Right Now, what emotion am I feeling?" Always answer out loud and write your answers in the allotted space
"I am feeling _____."

"Right Now, what emotion am I feeling?" Always answer out loud and write your answers in the allotted space
"I am feeling _____."

"Right Now, what emotion am I feeling?" Always answer out loud and write your answers in the allotted space
"I am feeling _____."

"Right Now, what emotion am I feeling?" Always answer out loud and write your answers in the allotted space
"I am feeling _____."

"Right Now, what emotion am I feeling?" Always answer out loud and write your answers in the allotted space
"I am feeling _____."

"Right Now, what emotion am I feeling?" Always answer out loud and write your answers in the allotted space
"I am feeling _____."

What physical activities did you participate in today?

_____

_____

_____

_____

_____

_____

_____

_____

_____

_____

_____

_____

_____

_____

_____

Send an e-mail to *workbook@zeropainnow.com* confirming you performed your tasks along with any updates about your progress. This will help you stay accountable for your daily actions. Also, some of the entries are reviewed by Adam and other trained *Zero Pain Now* staff who may reply to you with valuable feedback.

DAY 25

You are almost done with your program. What relationships or circumstances in your life that you need to eradicate or change today to reduce your stress, tension, anger or rage? What specifically will you do?

_____

_____

_____

_____

_____

_____

_____

_____

_____

_____

_____

_____

_____

_____

_____

_____

Spend at least 15 consecutive minutes asking yourself the following question:

"Right Now, what emotion am I feeling?" Always answer out loud and write your answers in the allotted space
"I am feeling _____."

"Right Now, what emotion am I feeling?" Always answer out loud and write your answers in the allotted space
"I am feeling _____."

"Right Now, what emotion am I feeling?" Always answer out loud and write your answers in the allotted space
"I am feeling _____."

"Right Now, what emotion am I feeling?" Always answer out loud and write your answers in the allotted space
"I am feeling _____."

"Right Now, what emotion am I feeling?" Always answer out loud and write your answers in the allotted space
"I am feeling _____."

"Right Now, what emotion am I feeling?" Always answer out loud and write your answers in the allotted space
"I am feeling _____."

"Right Now, what emotion am I feeling?" Always answer out loud and write your answers in the allotted space
"I am feeling _____."

"Right Now, what emotion am I feeling?" Always answer out loud and write your answers in the allotted space
"I am feeling _____."

"Right Now, what emotion am I feeling?" Always answer out loud and write your answers in the allotted space
"I am feeling _____."

"Right Now, what emotion am I feeling?" Always answer out loud and write your answers in the allotted space
"I am feeling _____."

"Right Now, what emotion am I feeling?" Always answer out loud and write your answers in the allotted space
"I am feeling _____."

"Right Now, what emotion am I feeling?" Always answer out loud and write your answers in the allotted space
"I am feeling _____."

"Right Now, what emotion am I feeling?" Always answer out loud and write your answers in the allotted space
"I am feeling _____."

"Right Now, what emotion am I feeling?" Always answer out loud and write your answers in the allotted space
"I am feeling _____."

"Right Now, what emotion am I feeling?" Always answer out loud and write your answers in the allotted space
"I am feeling _____."

"Right Now, what emotion am I feeling?" Always answer out loud and write your answers in the allotted space
"I am feeling _____."

"Right Now, what emotion am I feeling?" Always answer out loud and write your answers in the allotted space
"I am feeling _____."

"Right Now, what emotion am I feeling?" Always answer out loud and write your answers in the allotted space
"I am feeling _____."

"Right Now, what emotion am I feeling?" Always answer out loud and write your answers in the allotted space
"I am feeling _____."

"Right Now, what emotion am I feeling?" Always answer out loud and write your answers in the allotted space
"I am feeling _____."

"Right Now, what emotion am I feeling?" Always answer out loud and write your answers in the allotted space
"I am feeling _____."

"Right Now, what emotion am I feeling?" Always answer out loud and write your answers in the allotted space
"I am feeling _____."

"Right Now, what emotion am I feeling?" Always answer out loud and write your answers in the allotted space
"I am feeling _____."

"Right Now, what emotion am I feeling?" Always answer out loud and write your answers in the allotted space
"I am feeling _____."

"Right Now, what emotion am I feeling?" Always answer out loud and write your answers in the allotted space
"I am feeling _____."

How were you physical today?

_____

_____

_____

_____

_____

_____

_____

_____

_____

_____

_____

_____

_____

_____

_____

Send an e-mail to *workbook@zeropainnow.com* confirming you performed your tasks along with any updates about your progress. This will help you stay accountable for your daily actions. Also, some of the entries are reviewed by Adam and other trained *Zero Pain Now* staff who may reply to you with valuable feedback.

DAY 26

Today just remember to think psychologically. Focus on your emotions. What emotions are you feeling? Spend the entire day paying attention to your emotions.

Send an e-mail to *workbook@zeropainnow.com* confirming you performed your tasks along with any updates about your progress. This will help you stay accountable for your daily actions. Also, some of the entries are reviewed by Adam and other trained *Zero Pain Now* staff who may reply to you with valuable feedback.

DAY 27

What has changed for you? List all the ways that you have changed your life for the better in the last month.

If you're not smiling, you haven't written everything.

_____

_____

_____

_____

_____

_____

_____

_____

_____

_____

_____

_____

Send an e-mail to *workbook@zeropainnow.com* confirming you performed your tasks along with any updates about your progress. This will help you stay accountable for your daily actions. Also, some of the entries are reviewed by Adam and other trained *Zero Pain Now* staff who may reply to you with valuable feedback.

DAY 28

You did it! You dedicated yourself to changing and creating a life with physical freedom.

Go to **http://www.zeropainow.com/videoday28** for a special message for you from Adam.

To continue your progress you must remember to think psychologically and focus on your emotions.

You are in control of your brain.

Ending your cycle of pain is quick for some people and takes longer for others. Wherever you are is fine. Anyone who takes longer can still be successful in banishing your pain. Commit to your process. Continue to look inside and focus on emotions. Keep moving forward......................

4240248R00057

Made in the USA
San Bernardino, CA
07 September 2013